I0464297

# GUIDE
## TO COMMON
## **CROSS** COVER
## CALLS

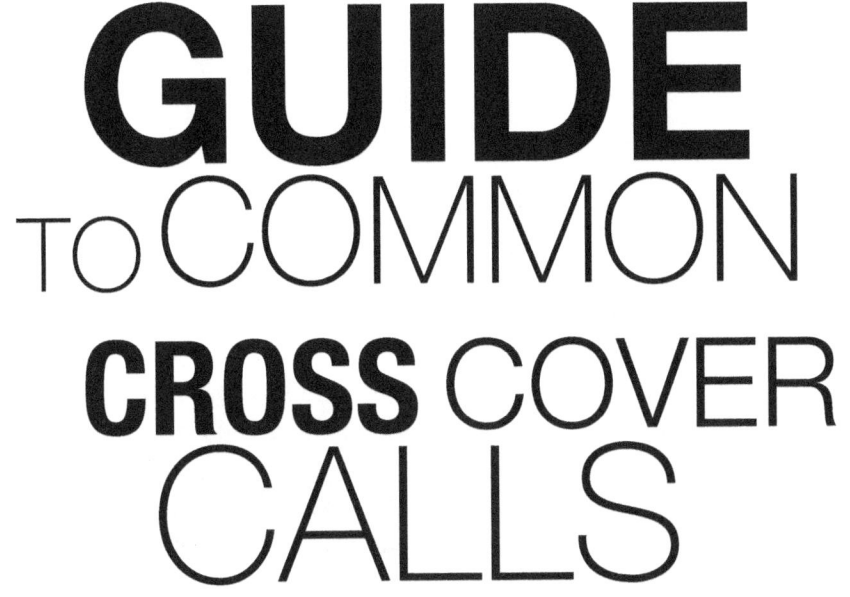

# GUIDE
## TO COMMON
## **CROSS** COVER
## CALLS

**Sunita Sharma MD, PhD**

Copyright © 2014 by Sunita Sharma MD, PhD.

ISBN:        Softcover            978-1-4836-7843-6
             eBook                978-1-4836-7844-3

All rights reserved. No part of this book may be reproduced or transmitted in any form or by any means, electronic or mechanical, including photocopying, recording, or by any information storage and retrieval system, without permission in writing from the copyright owner.

This guide is intended to assist you in taking care of some very common cross-cover calls especially during the first few months of internship. This is by no means a comprehensive guide but just to get you started. Please use additional sources to assist you in management of an individual patient. Always call your senior resident when you need help.

This book was printed in the United States of America.

Rev. date: 01/14/2014

**To order additional copies of this book, contact:**
Xlibris LLC
1-888-795-4274
www.Xlibris.com
Orders@Xlibris.com
137217

# Acknowledgements

I would like to extend my sincere thanks to Dr. Rajendra Potluri and Dr. Leonid Vilenski, Department of Hospital Internal Medicine, Sanford Health, Fargo for their expert suggestions.

# General rules for cross-cover

- Your aim is to take care of patient for the particular emergency situation, not to figure out all other chronic medical conditions

- Go see the patient if chest pain, hypoxia, fall with potential injuries, seizures or when in doubt

- When you go see the patient, write short progress note and update the primary team next day

- Follow up on labs/imaging you ordered on cross cover

- When writing medications specially for insomnia or pain, write for one time doses and avoid standing orders

- **When in doubt—call your senior resident/attending physician**

# Encephalopathy /Altered mental status

- Is this a new change? Delirium—acute fluctuation
- Ensure adequate airway, breathing and circulation
- Recent/new medications
- Check vitals, do neurological exam
- Review Labs: cardiac enzymes, electrolytes, any positive cultures
- Consider checking blood sugar, oxygen saturation, ABG, ammonia, TSH
- Consider checking non-contrast head CT (in presence of headache, vomiting, focal neurological signs)
- Try naloxone (Narcan), usually 0.4-1.2 mg IV, if there is any possibility of narcotic overdose
- If elderly person is agitated/sundowning
  - o Reorient frequently
  - o Have family member at bed side
  - o Assess need for sitter, bed alarm
  - o Restraints (last resort)
- Medications for agitated delirium
  - o Haloperidol (Haldol) 1-2 mg IV (IM only when cannot give IV)
  - o Olanzepine (Zyprexa) 2.5 mg IV/IM/PO q6h
  - o Avoid Benzodiazepines in elderly (except in alcohol withdrawal)

# Seizures

- Go to bedside to determine if patient still actively seizing
- Assess airway, breathing and circulation
- Give oxygen, Call anesthesia/RRT/code
- Place patient in lateral decubitus position with a suction device
- Check electrolytes (sodium, calcium), glucose, BUN
- Think of the cause—hypoxia, alcohol withdrawal, drug intoxication, cerebrovascular episode, head trauma
- Consider CT scan/EEG
- Consider drug screen if clinical history suggests recreational drug use
- Give thiamine 100 mg IV first, then 50 ml of 50% Dextrose (if alcohol withdrawal is a consideration)
- Antipyretics/cooling blankets for fever
- **Lorazepam (Ativan) 0.1 mg/kg IV at 2 mg/min**
- If no IV access—diazepam rectal gel (15-20 mg) or midazolam 5 mg IM or fosphenytoin 20 mg/kg IM
- If seizures continue:
  - o Load Phenytoin 15-20 mg/kg IV in 3 divided doses at 50 mg/min (usually 1g total) or Fosphenytoin 20 mg/kg IV at 150 mg/min
  - o If still seizing >30 min, patient is in status epilepticus—consider transfer to ICU for possible intubation or Phenobarbital

Sunita Sharma MD, PhD

# Insomnia

- Ask the patient what is keeping them awake—anxiety/pain/cough
- Shut off the lights and turn off the television
- Avoid caffeinated beverage
- Ask patient if they have used something in past that helped—give the same
- Medications that can be used
    o Trazodone 25-50 mg PO x 1 (do not affect blood pressure; preferred in elderly)
    o Zolpidem (Ambien) 5-10 mg PO x 1 (elderly 2.5 mg)
    o Temazepam 7.5-15 mg PO QHS
    o Diphenydramine (Benadryl) 25 mg PO QHS (Avoid in older patients due to anticholinergic effects)
- Other medications with benadryl
    o Acetaminophen-Diphenhydramine (500/25-Tylenol PM)
    o Acetaminophen-Diphenhydramine (500/38-Excedrin PM)
- Write only one time doses for your cross-cover (No standing PRN orders)
- Use lower doses in the elderly and liver failure patients.

# Falls

- Go see the patient if they sustain a fall in the hospital

- Find out the circumstances of fall

- Check vital signs

- Examine patient—neurological status, any injuries sustained from the fall, evidence of fractures

- Check recent labs, EKG, telemetry

- Look at medications as possible cause of fall

- If head trauma/altered mental status—consider CT head, several neuro-checks

- Any injuries—Consider X-rays to rule out fractures

- Place patient on fall precautions

- Assess need for assisted device

# Cough

- Make sure that it is not new acute onset cough related to aspiration

- Ask if it started after patient choked on food—if yes then keep patient NPO till swallow evaluation obtained

- Check oxygen saturation

- If cough with fever or shortness of breath, suspect infections

- Any history suggestive of upper respiratory infection/ asthma/GERD

- If chronic cough and patient wants something for symptomatic relief then,

  o Expectorant—Guaifenesin/Dextromethorphan 10-30 mg PO Q4H PRN

  o Benzonatate capsule (Tessalon Perles), 100 mg PO TID

  o If non-productive then cough suppressant— Codeine Phosphate 10-20 mg PO Q4H PRN (avoid codeine in patient with altered mental status or on pain medications)

# Shortness of breath and hypoxia

- Go see the patient
- Ask if onset of dyspnea acute or gradual
- Focused history and exam including vitals
- Consider cardiac versus pulmonary
- Associated symptoms—chest pain, positional change in pain
- Check your sign-out for any possible causes like CHF, pneumonia, COPD
- Consider ABG, CXR, EKG, troponin, pro-BNP
- Don't miss acute myocardial infarction, aspiration and pneumothorax
- Don't miss PE (hypoxia and tachycardia with relatively normal chest X-ray)—consider CT scan of chest PE protocol
- Emergent echocardiogram if suspect tamponade
- Consider need of diuretics, discontinuing IV fluids, oxygen to maintain saturation
- Call respiratory therapist—consider nebulizer therapy, BPAP

# Shortness of breath and hypoxia

## Supplemental Oxygen

- Nasal canula: for mild desaturations. Use humidified if giving more than >2L
- Face mask/Ventimask: offers up to 55% $FIO_2$
- Non-rebreather: offers up to 100% $FIO_2$
- BPAP: good for COPD and CHF

  (Not for patients with altered mental status)

  o Start settings at: IPAP 10 and EPAP 5, $FiO_2$ 100 %.

  o IPAP helps overcome work of breathing and helps to change $PCO_2$

  o EPAP helps change $PO_2$

# Anxiety

- Discuss with patient to find out what is causing anxiety—medical condition, financial or social issues
- Is there any history of generalized anxiety disorders or patient takes any medications at home
- Concern regarding substance abuse/withdrawal leading to anxiety
- Restart their home medications if needed especially if patient takes benzodiazepines on a regular basis
- If patient continues to remain anxious—try alprazolam (Xanax) 0.25-0.5 mg PO or lorazepam (Ativan) 0.5-1 mg PO/IV

# Chest Pain

- Go see the patient

- Focused history and exam

- Consider—cardiac or pulmonary etiologies

- Don't miss aortic dissection—consider immediate surgical consultation

- If spontaneous pneumothorax (16 gauge needle second intercostal space in mid-clavicular line)

- If history of CAD/appears cardiac—12-lead EKG, troponin, Nitro SL/spray, aspirin, oxygen

- If hypoxia and tachycardia—consider PE

- If pleuritic chest pain and shortness of breath—consider respiratory causes—get Chest X-ray (eg. Pneumothorax)

- If suspect gastroesophageal reflux—aluminium hydroxide (Maalox) works faster than proton pump inhibitor or H2 receptor antagonist

    o Aluminium hydroxide (Maalox) antacid 30 ml PO Q6H PRN (avoid in renal failure)

- If reproducible on palpation suggesting musculoskeletal in origin—Acetaminophen (Tylenol) (avoid NSAIDs in hospitalized patients)

- Call senior resident/chief resident if patient unstable

# Hypertension

- Check previous blood pressures and trend in blood pressure
- Patient anxious, in pain or withdrawing from alcohol
- Symptoms—chest pain, shortness of breath, altered mental status, headache—<u>urgency/emergency</u>
- If tearing chest pain radiating to back—consider aortic dissection
- Consider CT scan of head if focal neurological deficit to rule out cerebrovascular episode
- Any blood pressure medications on board?
- Treat high blood pressure in hospitalized patient only if symptomatic or persistently elevated
- Consider increasing dosages of home anti-hypertensives
- If heart rate can tolerate
  - o Labetalol 100 mg PO or 10 mg IV Q4H
- If heart rate on lower side or risk of bradycardia
  - o Hydralazine 25 mg PO or 10-20 mg IV Q4H (Avoid in patients with coronary artery disease)

# Hypotension

- Is patient symptomatic—drowsy, confused, decreased urine output, signs of hypoperfusion
- Look at the blood pressure trend, recheck to confirm
- Be aware that patients with cirrhosis, CHF—BPs tend to be lower—no intervention needed if asymptomatic
- Is patient post-procedure that required anesthesia?
- Consider stopping anti-hypertensives and diuretics
- Check if any hypovolemia due to bleeding/ diarrhea/vomiting
    - o Try saline bolus 500-1000 ml
    - o Make sure that patient can tolerate fluids and does not have systolic heart failure
- Consider serial hemoglobin if bleeding suspected and transfuse blood PRN
- Consider sepsis if fever, tachycardia
    - o Lactic acid, blood cultures and empiric antibiotics
- Possible adrenal insufficiency
    - o Check cortisol/ACTH levels, electrolytes
    - o Replace volume rapidly
    - o Hydrocortisone 50-100 mg IV Q6H
- If anaphylactic shock with SOB, wheeze
    - o Epinehprine, diphenhydramine (Benadryl), oxygen

# Telemetry

- First make sure patient is stable hemodynamically—occasional PVCs or PACs are non-alarming

- **If associated symptoms (chest pain, dyspnea, dizziness, syncope, confusion) or hyptension present—needs immediate action**

- Is this first episode or happened before

- Check patient's medications—digoxin, diuretics, other anti-arrhythmics, bronchodilators

# Telemetry

## Tachyarrhythmias

- Sinus arrhythmia—normal variant
- Premature atrial contraction (PAC)
  - Seen with history of tobacco, alcohol or caffeine use
- Premature ventricular contraction (PVC)
  - Seen with infection, myocardial infarction, tobacco, alcohol or caffeine use
- Atrial flutter/fibrillation with Rapid Ventricular Rate
  - Seen with valvular heart disease, myocardial infarction, alcohol intoxication, thyrotoxicosis
  - Rate control (beta-blocker—metoprolol or calcium channel blocker diltiazem or digoxin if systolic heart failure/blood pressure low)
  - Consider anti-arrhythmic (amiodarone)
- Supra Ventricular Tachycardia/SVT with aberrancy
  - Vagal maneuver (avoid carotid massage in elderly)
  - Adenosine 6-12 mg IV
- Ventricular Tachycardia
  - Check magnesium and potassium level
  - Keep magnesium > 2 and potassium > 4
  - Give magnesium for polymorphic VT/torsades de pointes
  - Consider amiodarone/procainamide
  - If sustained > 30 seconds—call RRT/Code

# Telemetry

## Bradyarrhythmias

- Assess airway breathing and circulation—give oxygen, monitor blood pressure

- Any associated symptoms—fatigue, syncope, nausea, dyspnea, chest pain, decreased urine output, altered mental status

- Get 12 lead EKG, serum electrolytes, arterial blood gases, serum drug levels

- Consider SA node dysfunction, inferior wall infarctions, drug effect, increased intracranial pressure (cushing's reflex), malfunctioning pacemaker

- AV block: 1st (prolonged PR), 2nd (prolonging PR with drop QRS) or 3rd degree (PR not prolonged with drop QRS)
    - o Hold beta blockers, calcium channel blockers
    - o If Mobitz type 2 or complete heart block
        - Consider Atropine 0.5 mg IV x3 doses (if symptomatic sinus bradycardia)
        - Call cardiology for possible temporary pacing
        - If digoxin toxicity—Digoxin antibody

# Oliguria/Anuria

- Oliguria is defined as urine output 100-400 ml/24h or <30 ml/hr

- Consider possible conditions—shock, hypotentions, obtruction

- Get vitals, ask for bladder scan

- If volume > 200 ml—straight cath

- If already catheterized flush Foley catheter to ensure patency

- If volume < 200 ml—fluid challenge (normal saline), check blood pressure

- Consider using diuretics

- Check if patient is in renal failure—electrolytes for hyperkalemia, uremia, metabolic acidosis

- If acute renal failure—consider pre-renal (hypovolemia), renal or post-renal (obstruction) etiologies

- Consider need for dialysis

    o Note: Indications for Emergent Dialysis

        ▪ A—Acidosis, refractory

        ▪ E—Electrolytes (refractory hyperkalemia)

        ▪ I—Intoxication

        ▪ O—Overload (fluid overload, refractory)

        ▪ U—Uremic pericarditis

# Abdominal Pain

- Go to the bedside.

- Assess vitals, rapidity of onset, location, quality and severity of pain; associated symptoms (nausea, vomiting, constipation)

- Don't miss AAA, bowel ischemia or perforation (guarding and rigidity), cholangitis, appendicitis, cholecystitis, pancreatitis

- Could be as simple as gastritis or radiating pain of nephrolithiasis

- Make sure it is not atypical presentation of anginal pain

- Consider DKA if patient has history of diabetes

- Consider

    o X-ray abdomen (flat and upright) to rule out free air under diaphragm/ bowel obstruction

    o Lipase, amylase (pancreatitis)

    o CBC, electrolytes, creatinine, BUN, lactic acid (bowel ischemia)

    o Right upper quadrant ultrasound, liver function test (cholecystitis)

    o Consider CT scan of abdomen if other tests inconclusive

    o Consider 12-lead EKG if concern that pain could possibly be cardiac in origin

# Nausea and Vomiting

- Check vitals

- Assess patient's volume status—need for IV fluids

- Rule out bowel obstruction (abdominal X-ray)

- Think of common causes—pain medications, gastritis

- Consider serious causes—raised intracranial pressure (hypertension and bradycardia), appendicitis, pancreatitis, sepsis (fever)

- Consider GI bleed if blood/coffee ground vomitus

- Depending on suspected etiologies—consider checking labs (CBC, electrolytes, liver function test, lipase, amylase)

- Common anti-nausea medications

  o Ondansetron (Zofran) 4-8 mg PO/IV Q6H PRN

  o Metoclopramide (Reglan) 5-10 mg PO/IV Q6H PRN (Can cause dystonic reactions)

  o Promethazine (Phenargan) 12.5-25 mg PO/PR/IM Q6H PRN or Prochlorperazine (Compazine) 5-10 mg IV/PO/IM Q6H PRN/ suppository 25 mg BID (caution in elderly as can cause extrapyramidal symptoms)

  o Droperidol (Inapsine) 2-5 mg IV Q6H PRN

  o Hydroxyzine 50 mg IM/PO Q4H PRN

# Diarrhea

- Check vitals
- If fever (infection), hypotenstion (hypovolemia), abdominal pain or blood in stool (ischemic bowel, inflammatory bowel disease, invasive infection)
- Make sure patient is not dehydrated, consider IV fluids
- Consider discontinuing laxatives/stool softner
- Send stool for C. difficle PCR
- Do not miss C. difficle colitis with dilated colon (toxic megacolon)—consider X-ray abdomen
- Check electrolytes and replace appropriately
- Lactose free diet
- Only if not infectious diarrhea
  - o Loperamide (Imodium) 4 mg then 2 mg PO with each bowel movement, max 16 mg/day
  - o Bismuth subsalicylate (Pepto-Bismol) 30 ml PO Q6H PRN

# Constipation

- Abdomen distended, tender or associated with nausea and vomiting—consider bowel obstructions
- If post-surgical—consider paralytic ilieus

**If no nausea/vomiting, abdominal pain, or fecal impaction**

- Stool Softeners (detergents)
  - o Sodium docusate (Colace) 100 mg PO BID—works for prevention not for treatment
- Stimulants (in acute constipation)
  - o Senna 1-2 tablets BID PRN
  - o Bisacodyl (Dulcolax) 10-15 mg PO Q4H PRN
- Osmotics
  - o Polyethylene glycol (Miralax/Glycolax) 17 gm in 8oz water BID—best
  - o Lactulose/ 30 ml (20 gm) PO Q6H until bowel movement (preferred in liver disease)
  - o Magnesium citrate 150-300 ml PO BID
  - o Milk of magnesia 15-30 ml PO BID (avoid in renal disease)
- Enemas
  - o Tap water
  - o Sodium biphosphate (fleet)

**<u>Avoid Fleet Enemas in patients with renal disease or CHF</u>**

# Heart burn/GERD/Indigestion

- Ensure that head of the bed is elevated, avoid aspiriation
- Medications that can be used
    - Famotidine (Pepcid) 20 mg PO/IV BID
    - Ranitidine (Zantac) 150 mg PO/IV TID
    - Omeprazole (Prilosec) 40 mg PO daily
    - Lansoprazole (Protonix) 40 mg IV daily
- Stress Ulcer Prophylaxis (not required routinely on general floor)
- Indigestion
    - Aluminium hydroxide (Maalox) antacid 30 ml PO Q6H PRN (avoid in renal failure)
    - Calcium carbonate (Tums) 500 mg PO TID

# Pain Management

Please do appropriate work-up as needed depending on type, location and severity of pain

- <u>Mild Pain</u>
    - o Acetaminophen (Tylenol) 325-650 mg PO every Q4H PRN (do not exceed 4 g/day), scheduled works better than PRN
    - o Avoid acetaminophen with codeine (Tylenol # 3) 30/300 mg PO Q6H (addicting, less pain control, more nausea and vomiting)
    - o Ibuprofen 200 mg PO Q6H (Avoid NSAIDs in renal failure, CHF, resistant hypertension, peptic ulcer disease)
- <u>Moderate Pain</u>
    - o Hydrocodone/acetaminophen (Narco/Lortab/ Vicodin) 5/325 mg PO Q4H
    - o Oxycodone/acetaminophen (Percocet) 5/325 mg PO Q4H
    - o Oxycodone immediate release 5 mg PO Q4H
    - o Oxycodone sustained release 10 mg PO Q12H
    - o Tramadol 50 mg PO Q6H

# Pain Management

- Severe Pain

    o Morphine 10-20 mg PO Q4H

    o Hydromorphone (Dilaudid) 0.5-1 mg IV Q3H

    o Hydromorhphone (Dilaudid) 2 mg PO Q4H

    o Fentanyl 25 mcg IV Q1H (short acting—works better as PCA)

Other options:

- Ketorolac (Toradol) 15 mg IV Q6H (for inflammatory pain, do not exceed > 6days, avoid in patients with renal failure)

- Fentanyl patch 12-25 mcg/h (change every 72 hours—not for acute pain relief)

- Lidocaine patch 5% (12 hours on and 12 hours off for localized nerve pain)

- Neuropathic pain

    o Amitriptyline 25 mg PO QHS

    o Gabapentin (Neurontin) 300 mg PO BID

- Muscle relaxants

    o Cyclobenzaparine (Flexeril) 5-10 mg PO TID

    o Metaxalone (Skelaxin) 800 mg PO TID

# Pain Management

Opioid Equianalgesic Dose

| Opioid | IV | PO/PR | Duration (h) |
|---|---|---|---|
| Morphine | 5 | 15 | 3-4 |
| Long acting morphine | NA | 15 | 8-12 |
| Oxycodone | NA | 10 | 3-4 |
| Long acting oxycodone | NA | 10 | 8-12 |
| Hydromorphone | 0.75 | 4 | 3-4 |
| Codeine | 50 | 100 | 3-4 |
| Hydrocodone | NA | 15 | 3-4 |

Opioid dose equivalent to 25 mcg/h fentanyl patch

| Drug | Oral | IV |
|---|---|---|
| Morphine | 45 mg/24h | 15 mg/24h |
| Hydromorphone | 10 mg/24h | 2 mg/24h |

Note:

Fentanyl transdermal patch is not for acute pain

Hydromorphone and fentanyl preferred over codeine, morphine and oxycodone in liver and kidney disease

# Fever

- New fever in hospital suggest hospital acquired infection

- Concerning if patient immunocompromised or neutropenic

- Any indwelling catheters or lines present

- Any obvious source of infection—urinary symptoms, cough, diarrhea

- Any recent procedures or blood transfusion

- Examine skin for cellulitis/skin lesions and joints for arthritis

- Check blood cultures, urine analysis with reflex to culture

- Consider sputum gram stain and culture if patient is coughing

- Chest X-Ray if indicated
    - o  PA and lateral preferable
    - o  Portable if patient unstable

- To bring temperature down, use acetaminophen 650 mg PO/rectal Q4H PRN and cooling blankets

- Consider empiric antibiotics if patient hemodynamically unstable with possible infectious source for fever

# Rash/Pruritus

- Examine skin for localized or systemic rash

- Make sure there is no signs of anaphylaxis, check vitals

- Stop the offending agent, if known

- If anaphylactic reaction (shortness of breath, wheezing, urticarial rash—epinephrine 0.5 mg IM, hydrocortisone 250 mg IV

- If Vancomycin—slow down the rate of infusion

- Symptomatic treatment for pruritus

  o Benadryl 25-50 mg PO/IV Q6H PRN/prior to infusion

  o Hydroxyzine (Atarax) 25 mg PO Q6H PRN

  o Fexofenadine (Allegra) non sedating—180 mg PO daily (lower doses in elderly patient)

- Topical agents

  o Camphor 0.5% and Menthol 0.5% (Sarna lotion)

  o Capsaicin 0.075%

  o Doxepin 5% cream Q4H

- Refractory pruritus

  o Doxepin 25 mg PO daily (for short period of time)

- If contact/eczematous dermatitis—consider emollient or topical steroids

- If uremia or cholestasis—consider cholestyramine

# Fungal infection

- Skin—Terbinafine (Lamisil) or Butenafine (Lotrimin) cream to affected area TID and PRN
- Skin—under breast/groin areas—Nystatin powder/cream (100,000 units/g) to affected area TID and PRN
- Vaginal candidiasis
    - o Miconazole (Monistat) cream vaginally QHS x 3 nights
    - o Fluconazole (Diflucan) 150 mg x 1 dose
- Oral thrush—Nystatin 5 ml QID swish and swallow x 5 days

# Blood transfusion reactions

- If fever (self-limiting febrile transfusion reaction)
  - o Decrease rate of transfusion
  - o Give Tylenol 650 mg PO
  - o Meperidine 20-50 mg IV can be given for shakes/ chills
- If severe hemolytic reaction suspected (hypotension, fever, tachycardia)
  - o Stop transfusion immediately
  - o Send blood that is being transfused and patient's blood for cross match,
  - o Check Coombs' test, CBC, DIC panel, total bilirubin, electrolyte panel
  - o Rehydration with IV fluids
  - o Monitor renal function and electrolytes
  - o Keep UOP > 100 ml/h
- If severe, non-hemolytic reaction suspected (anaphylactic, wheezing, SOB, temperature >104oF)
  - o Stop transfusion, send bag for repeat cross-match
  - o Diphenhydramine (Benadryl) 25-50 mg PO/IV
  - o Consider Hydrocortisone 250-500 mg IV
  - o Consider epinephrine 0.5-1.0 ml (1:1000) IM
- If volume overload
  - o Decrease rate of transfusion
  - o Furesomide (Lasix) 20-40 mg IV
  - o Chest X-ray to rule out Transfusion Related Acute Lung Injury (TRALI)

# Blood Sugar Management

- Remember first rule—avoid hypoglycemia

- To avoid morning hypoglycemia—consider bed time snacks and no night time insulin correction dose

- If blood sugars are high overnight, consider adjusting insulin only if blood sugars > 400 and you are concerned about DKA (nausea, vomiting and abdominal pain)

- Do not increase from low to medium to high dose supplemental insulin in patients with history of hypoglycemia

- Avoid insulin stacking in patients with renal disease

- Review trends in previous blood sugars and amount of insulin patient received in last 24 hours before making adjustments

- If patient having blood sugars towards low normal and is eating—do not reduce long-acting basal insulin (Lantus/ Levemir)

# Restarting Diet

- Any procedures done today
  - o Can patient resume his previous diet
  - o Did GI/Surgery/IR recommended diet in procedure notes
  - o Is patient alert awake to eat
- Does patient need bedside swallow screen (any concern for dysphagia)
- Any procedures planned for tomorrow
- If no concern and primary team has just forgot to start diet/ procedure completed, then go ahead and start diet based on chronic co-morbid conditions
  - o Heart healthy, diabetic or renal
  - o Dysphagia soft (nearly regular textures with the exception of very hard, sticky or crunchy foods)
  - o Dysphagia mechanical soft (moist, soft textured, and easily formed into a round mass)
  - o Dysphagia puree (pudding-like foods, no coarse textures, raw fruits, vegetables or nuts allowed)
  - o Thin/Honey thick/nectar thick liquid

# Hyperkalemia

- Check vitals, urine output, 12-lead EKG
- Repeat potassium levels (to rule of hemolysis of sample)
- Discontinue potassium supplements, ACE inhibitors, potassium sparing diuretics
- Mild (K<6)
    - o Furosemide (Lasix) 40-80 mg IV
    - o Sodium Polystrene (Kayexalate) 30 g in 50 ml of 20% sorbitol PO/PR
- Moderate (K 6-7)
    - o Sodium bicarbonate 50 mEq IV over 5 min
    - o Dextrose50 (50 g) + insulin 10 units IV over 15 min
    - o Albuterol 10-20 mg nebulized over 15 min
- Severe (K>7) or EKG changes (peaked T-waves)
    - o Calcium chloride 10% (central line) 5-10 ml or calcium gluconate 10% (peripheral line) 15-30 ml over 2-5 min
    - o Avoid calcium in suspected digitalis toxicity
    - o Also use sodium bicarbonate or dextrose + insulin as above to redistribute and then sodium polystrene (Kayexalate) and Furosemide (Lasix) to excrete potassium
    - o Consider dialysis if refractory hyperkalemia

# Hypernatremia

- Check patient's mental status

- Review intake and output (hypovolemia/ dehydration)

- Consider diabetes insipidus (polyuria), hyperaldosteronism

- If patient is on tube feeds—ensure free water flushes

- Check urine sodium and urine osmolality

- If acute increase in serum sodium due to hypovolemia/dehydration then give normal saline

- If euvolemic hypernatremia—give 0.45% normal saline (do not correct sodium level too rapidly)

- Calculate free water deficit and give ½ in first 12 hours and then other ½ in next 24 hours

# Electrolyte Replacement

General rules

- Keep potassium > 4 if arrhythmias

- Keep magnesium > 2 if arrhythmias

- Be cautious when replacing potassium and magnesium in patients with end stage renal disease

- Discuss with nephrologist if patient is on dialysis

- Prefer oral replacement over IV whenever possible

- Correct hypomagnesemia in patients with hypokalemia and hypocalcemia

# Hypokalemia

- Potassium 3-3.5 and creatinine < 2.0

If can take orally

- o Potassium chloride 40 mEq twice daily x 2 doses
- o If patient have trouble swallowing try smaller tablets of 10 mEq or try potassium chloride solution (but solution can cause nausea)

If cannot take orally

- o Potassium chloride 20 mEq IV with 20 mg lidocaine over 2 hours

- Potassium 2.5-3.0 and creatinine < 2.0
  - o Potassium chloride 40 mEq IV with 20 mg lidocaine over 2 hours

- Potassium 2.5-3.0 and creatinine > 2.0
  - o Potassium chloride 20 mEq IV with 20 mg lidocaine over 2 hours

- If K 3-3.5—every 10mEq of potassium raises K by 0.1
- If K < 3—every 20mEq of potassium raises K by 0.1

# Hypomagnesemia

- Magnesium 1.5-1.8

    o If can take orally then Magnesium oxide 500 mg 2-3 times a day

    o Avoid oral magnesium oxide in patients with diarrhea

    o Magnesium sulfate 2 g IV over 1 hour

- Magnesium < 1.5

    o Magnesium sulfate 4 g IV over 2 hours

# Hypocalcemia

- Ionized calcium less than 1.0 mmol/L or corrected calcium is low or symptomatic hypocalcemia
  - o Calcium gluconate (10%) 20 ml solution IV over 30 min
  - o If central line—calcium chloride (10%) 10 ml solution IV over 15 min
- Chronic hypocalcemia
  - o Calcium carbonate (Tums) 500 mg PO Q8H

# Hypophosphatemia

- Phosphorus < 2.5 and creatinine > 2.0 Or potassium > 4.0
    - NaPhos 40 mmoles IV over 4 hours (OK to give if elevated serum sodium)
    - If can take orally Neutraphos packet 2-3 times a day
- Phosphorus < 2.5 and creatinine < 2.0 and potassium < 4
    - Give KPhos 40 mmoles with 20 g of lidocaine IV over 6 hours
    - Do not need to use lidocaine if given by central line.

# Hyponatremia

- Find out if this is acute/chronic and new/old

- Patient symptomatic—anorexia, nausea, vomiting, altered mental status or seizures

- Check vitals, volume status

- Any evidence of renal disease, congestive heart failure, cirrhosis, nephrotic syndrome

- History suggestive of hypothyroidism, adrenal insufficiency

- Any medications—NSAIDs, SSRIs, diuretics

- Any central nervous system or pulmonary disease

- If hypovolemic hyponatremia

    o Normal saline IV

- If euvolemic hyponatremia/SIADH

    o Fluid restriction 800-1000 ml daily

- If hypervolemic hyponatremia

    o Treatment of underlying cause like congestive heart failure, nephrotic syndrome, cirrhosis or renal failure

- If acute hyponatremia with CNS symptoms/seizures

    o Normal saline with Furosemide

    o Hypertonic saline 3%

    o Correct rapidly till serum sodium 120-125, then slowly correct sodium level < 0.5mmol/L/h

# IV access

- Determine if IV access is necessary
    - o  Is patient NPO and may need IV fluids
    - o  Does patient need emergency IV medications
    - o  Consider if IV medications can be given orally
    - o  Are there discharge plans already for next day by primary team
- If IV access necessary—Call Flight team or anesthesia for difficult IV
- If nothing is working—PICC line
- If not an option (PICC line nurse not available, IR nurse can place PICC)—consider central venous access (ICU physicians)

# Leaving Against Medical Advice

- Go talk to the patient

- Determine if patient has capacity to make decision or not

- If not capacity then consider placing on hold till find about substitute consent

- If competent—try to understand why patient wants to leave AMA

- Explain to the patient the health risks involved going AMA

- Explain that when leaving AMA—may have problems with insurance coverage and medications

- Can try to contact the primary team member on phone for details

- Do formal discharge for the patient if patient stable to go

# Family/Patient wants to talk to the 'doctor'

- Get the information from nurse if there was anything specific patient or family wanted to talk about
- Check the sign-out sheet and briefly review chart
- Go visit with patient/family.
- Introduce yourself and tell them upfront that you are covering for emergencies so you may not be that familiar with the patient's case, but based on the sign-out by primary team and review of the chart you will try to answer their questions to best of your ability
- Try to answer questions the best you can and let family know that the primary doctor would be available next day to discuss more details

# Death

- Check for:
    - o Response to verbal or painful stimuli, pupillary reflex, respiration, heart sounds, carotid and femoral pulse)
- **Call time of death**
- Talk to the family in person, if not available then on phone
    - o Explain to them what happened
    - o Ask if they have any questions
    - o Ask if they would like someone from spiritual care to be called
    - o Let them know they may have time with the deceased
- Ask family if they would like an autopsy
- Medical Examiner will be called if:
    - o Patient hospitalized <24 hours
    - o Death associated with unusual circumstances (e.g. poisoning)
    - o Sudden death with no obvious explanation

# Pearls for admission

- Reconcile medications

- Address code status—where appropriate (discuss all aspects—chest compression, shocking the heart, breathing tube/intubation)

- Determine inpatient/outpatient/observation status

- Make sure you order DVT prophylaxis

- PRN orders for pain, nausea and vomiting, where needed

- Do not write daily weights, OT, PT in every patient—Think before you chose these orders to save resources where really required

  o Daily weights—CHF, ESRD dialysis patients

  o OT—elderly who need upper extremity exercises or cognitive assessment

  o PT—elderly who need mobilization/gait training (at risk of deconditioning) or assessment of independence for discharge planning

# Pearls for daily rounds

- Keep your patient list updated
- Always review chart systematically (vitals, intake output, labs, medications, etc)
- Make sure that nursing staff is aware that you are primary provider taking care of the patients
- Nursing staff reports are very important
- Questions to ask on every patient while rounding?
    o Discontinue/Adjust IV fluids
    o IV meds be changed to PO
    o Any home medications to be restarted
    o Discontinue Foley
    o Discontinue telemetry
    o Advance diet and increase activity
    o Is patient having bowel movements
    o Discharge plans—OT, PT, social services

# Pearls for discharge

- Discharge is a crucial process and you need to spend time on it
- Discharge plan starts on the day of admission
- Discuss discharge plans with your team well in advance—including medications and follow-up at the time of discharge
- Can make follow-up appointments day ahead of time
- Always update /sign-out to the provider for follow-up appointment
    - o  PCP/resident clinic
    - o  Provider from other facilities
    - o  Mid-level/MD at the nursing home
- Discharge summary should be done as soon as possible preferably same day of discharge (some hospitals/nursing homes require discharge summary to be completed before patient leaves the hospital)
- Clearly update patient and family with changes in medications, expected course of illness, new treatment plans and follow-up appointments

# Ordering Consults

- Make sure of the questions you want the consulting physician to answer
- Start with reason for consult when you call, so that the consulting physician is aware before giving the full history
- Always a good idea to have access to patient's chart if need to review to answer questions
- After hours/weekends consults—always call to make sure that consult has been received, you can still mention that patient can be seen next morning if no urgency
- Do not consult Psychiatry on every alcohol intoxications (Chemical dependency services can decide regarding psychiatry consult)
    - o Consult them if patient is suicidal, needs active management of psychiatric medications or is placed on hold

# MS-DRG Documentation

- Hypertension
    - o Accelerated = BP 160-179/100-119
    - o Malignant = BP > 180/120 + organ failure
    - o Benign = long standing hypertension not requiring acute treatment
    - o Secondary due to (specify)
- Morbid Obesity (if significant co-morbidity affecting hospitalization)
    - o Mention BMI (> 35 = morbid)
- Anemia
    - o Acute blood loss (> 20% drop in hemoglobin)
    - o Chronic blood loss (slow persistent escape of blood usually from chronic lesion in GI tract, gynecological or urological site)
    - o Acute on chronic blood loss
    - o Iron deficiency
    - o Unable to determine

# MS-DRG Documentation

Congestive heart failure

- Severity
    - o Acute—usually presents with worsening of dyspnea ± hypoxia ± pulmonary edema or cardiogenic shock of sudden onset. Requires hospitalization with acute treatment—IV diuretics, beta-blockers, ACE inhibitors
    - o Chronic—clinical syndrome that includes shortness of breath, dyspnea, cyanosis, fatigue and edema
    - o Acute on Chronic
- Nature
    - o Systolic—reduced ventricular EF (< 40%), a dilated left ventricle and multiple regional wall motion abnormalities
    - o Diastolic—normal EF (50-65%), (> 70%), a normal or small left ventricle, thickened ventricular walls with concentric hypertrophy and no segmental wall motion abnormalities.
    - o Combined—Combined systolic and diastolic dysfunction with an EF of (40-50%) have mixed heart failure

# MS-DRG Documentation

Respiratory Failure

- Acute Respiratory Failure =

    - Develops over minutes to hours

    - pH < 7.30 or > 7.5

    - pH < 7.35 $pCO_2$ > 50 and/or

    - $pO_2$ < 55; $sPO_2$ < 88% requiring > 28% of $FiO_2$

    - Use of accessory muscles; RR > 20; Cyanosis; Apparent distress; aggressive treatment

- COPD/Chronic Respiratory Failure =

    - Develops over minutes to hours

    - Requires ongoing home treatment to maintain stability. Identifying factors include: End stage COPD, continuous home oxygen required, continuous/scheduled home nebulizers use, chronic oral steroid use continuously, chronic home mechanical ventilation—invasive or on (BPAP)

- Pneumonia/Health Care Associated/Community Acquired

    o Clarify suspected organism or cause—probably aspiration/gram negative/MRSA pneumonia

# MS-DRG Documentation

- CKD
    - o Kidney disease with radiological abnormality, proteinuria, hematuria, GFR < 30 for > 3 months
    - o Check GFR for stages 1) > 90; 2) 60-89; 3) 30-59; 4)15-29; 5) < 15
- Acute Kidney Injury
    - o Abrupt decrease in serum creatinine > 0.3 mg/dl or serum creatinine > 1.5 x baseline or Urine output <0.5 ml/kg/h for > 6 hours (Stage 1: serum creatinine 1.5-19 x baseline or ≥ 0.3 mg/dl increase or urine output < 0.5 ml/kg/h for 6-12 hours; Stage 2: serum creatinine 2.0-2.9 x baseline or urine output < 0.5 ml/kg/h for ≥ 12 hours; Stage 3: serum creatinine 3.0 x baseline or serum creatinine ≥ 4.0 mg/dl or urine output < 0.3 ml/kg/h for ≥ 24 hours or anuria of ≥ 12 hours)
    - o Etiology—hypovolemia, contrast nephropathy, shock, toxins or ATN from other causes

# Useful Formulas

- Creatinine clearance (eGFR)

$$\frac{(140 - age) \times weight\ (kg)\ (\times\ 0.85\ for\ females)}{72 \times serum\ creatinine\ (mg/dL)}$$

- Anion Gap (Serum)

$$Na - (Cl + HCO_3)$$

- Anion Gap (Urine)

$$(Na + K) - Cl$$

- Corrected Total Calcium

$$[0.8 \times (normal\ albumin - patient\ albumin)] + Ca$$

- Corrected Sodium

$$Na + [(glucose-100) \times 0.016]$$

- Aa Gradient

$$[713 \times FiO_2) - (PaCO_2/0.8)] - PaO_2$$

- Osmolality

$$2 \times Na + glucose/18 + BUN/2.8$$

- Body Water Deficit (liters)

$$\frac{0.6 \times weight\ (kg) \times (patient\ Na - normal\ Na)}{Normal\ Na}$$

Sunita Sharma MD, PhD

# Useful Formulas

- Arterial Blood Gas Rule

    $\Delta$ 10 mm Hg $PaCO_2$ = $\Delta$ 0.08 pH

- Mean Arterial Pressure

    Diastolic BP + [(systolic BP-Diastolic BP)/3]

# Procedure-related Orders

- Cerebrospinal Fluid

    o  Tube 1 for cell count with differential

    o  Tube 2 for protein, glucose

    o  Tube 3 for bacterial culture, gram stain, If needed— TB stain, crypto stain, PCR for HSV, EBV, VZV, CMV, VDRL

    o  Tube 4 to hold for any further testing, if needed

- Pleural fluid

Get serum CBC, PTT, PT-INR, LDH, and Total Protein

    o  Cell count with differential, cytology

    o  Total protein, LDH, glucose (low in empyema and rheumatoid arthritis), amylase, and triglycerides (chylothorax), pH (send on ice; < 7.2 in empyema)

    o  Gram stain, culture (aerobic/anaerobic), Acid fast bacilli stain

Get follow-up Chest-Xray (to make sure no pneumothorax)

- Ascitic fluid

    o  Cell count and differential (neutrophil count for SBP), gram stain and culture, albumin, protein

    o  Consider glucose/LDH (if thinking perforation), amylase (if thinking pancreatitis), cytology, and Acid fast bacilli stain

# Disease Risk Score—TIMI (NSTEMI)

- In patients with Unstable Angina or NSTEMI the TIMI risk score predicts the % chance of all cause mortality, MI, or need for urgent revascularization within 14 days
- All Criteria are worth 1 point
  - Age ≥ 65 years
  - Known CAD lesion ≥ 50%
  - Aspirin use in last 7 days
  - Angina ≥ 2 episodes in last 24 hours
  - ST deviation ≥ 0.5 mm
  - Elevation of cardiac enzymes
  - Coronary artery disease risk factors ≥ 3

| Score | %Risk |
|-------|-------|
| 0-1   | 5     |
| 2     | 8     |
| 3     | 13    |
| 4     | 20    |
| 5     | 26    |
| 6-7   | 41    |

# Disease Risk Score—TIMI (STEMI)

- Age 75 years or older (+3)

- Age 65-74 years (+2)

- Systolic blood pressure < 100 mmHg (+3)

- Heart rate > 100 (+2)

- Killip Class II-IV (evidence of heart failure) (+2)

- Anterior ST-elevation or Left bundle branch block (+1)

- Diabetes, history of hypertension, or angina (+1)

- Weight < 67 kg (+1)

- Time to treatment > 4 hours (+1)

| Score | Predicted 30-day mortality (%) |
|-------|--------------------------------|
| 0 | 0.8 |
| 1 | 1.6 |
| 2 | 2.2 |
| 3 | 4.4 |
| 4 | 7.3 |
| 5 | 12.4 |
| 6 | 16.1 |
| 7 | 23.4 |
| 8 | 26.8 |
| >8 | 35.9 |

# Disease Risk Score—ABCD2 (Stroke)

ABCD2 Score (Predicts the % risk of stroke at 2, 7, and 90 days after a TIA)

- Age ≥ 60 years = 1 point
- Blood Pressure SBP >140 or DBP >90 = 1 point
- Clinical Presentation
    - o Unilateral Weakness = 2 points
    - o Speech Impairment without weakness = 1 point
- Duration of symptoms
    - o ≥ 60 minutes = 2 points
    - o 10-59 minutes = 1 point
- Diabetes Mellitus = 1 point

| % Risk | 2 days | 7 days | 90 days |
|--------|--------|--------|---------|
| Low <4 | 1.0 | 1.2 | 3.1 |
| Mod 4-5 | 4.1 | 5.9 | 9.8 |
| High > 5 | 8.1 | 11.7 | 17.8 |

# Disease Risk Score—CHADS2 Vasc (Stroke)

Should someone with atrial fibrillation be anticoagulated to prevent stroke

CHF—1

Hypertension—1

Age ≥ 75 years—2

DM—1

Stroke/TIA—2

Vascular disease (e.g. PVD, MI, aortic plaque)—1

Age 65-74 years—1

Sex category (i.e.female gender)—1

| Points | Annual stroke risk % |
|--------|----------------------|
| 0 | 0 |
| 1 | 1.3 |
| 2 | 2.2 |
| 3 | 3.2 |
| 4 | 4.0 |
| 5 | 6.7 |
| 6 | 9.8 |
| 7 | 9.6 (study had small sample size with this score, leading to more variability) |
| 8 | 6.7 (study had very small sample size) |
| 9 | 15.2 |

# Disease Risk Score—CURB 65 (Pneumonia)

CURB 65 score for pneumonia

- **C**onfusion of new onset

- **U**rea greater than 7 mmol/l (19 mg/dL)

- **R**espiratory rate of 30 breaths per minute or greater

- **B**lood pressure less than 90 mmHg systolic or diastolic blood pressure 60 mmHg or less

- Age **65** or older

| Points | Mortality risk at 30 days (%) |
|--------|-------------------------------|
| 0 | 0.6 |
| 1 | 3.2 |
| 2 | 13 |
| 3 | 17 |
| 4 | 41.5 |
| 5 | 57 |

# Disease Risk Score—Wells Criteria (DVT)

**Wells Criteria/scoring for DVT (possible score—2 to 9)**

- Lower limb trauma or surgery or immobilization in a plaster cast (+1)

- Bedridden for more than three days or surgery within the last four weeks (+1)

- Tenderness along line of femoral or popliteal veins (NOT just calf tenderness) (+1)

- Entire limb swollen (+1)

- Calf more than 3 cm bigger circumference, 10 cm below tibial tuberosity (+1)

- Pitting edema (+1)

- Dilated collateral superficial veins (non-varicose) (+1)

- Past history of confirmed DVT (+1)

- Malignancy (including treatment up to six months previously) (+1)

- Intravenous drug use (+3)

- Alternative diagnosis as more likely than DVT (-2)

**Pre-test Clinical probability of a DVT with score:**

- o   DVT "Likely" if Well's ≥ 2

- o   DVT "Unlikely" if Wells < 2

# Disease Risk Score—Wells Criteria (PE)

**Wells criteria / scoring for PE**

- Clinical Signs and Symptoms of DVT (+3)

- Alternative diagnosis is less likely than PE (+3)

- Heart Rate > 100 (+1.5)

- Immobilization at least 3 days, or surgery in the previous 4 weeks (+1.5)

- Previous, objectively diagnosed PE or DVT (+1.5)

- Hemoptysis (+1)

- Malignancy with treatment within 6 months, or palliative (+1)

**Pre-test clinical probability of a PE:**

- o Wells Score > 4 - PE likely. Consider diagnostic imaging.

- o Wells Score 4 or less - PE unlikely. Consider D-dimer to rule out PE

# Disease Risk Score—Ranson (Pancreatitis)

Ranson Criteria for predicting severity of acute pancreatitis

At admission or diagnosis:

- Age > 55 years
- White blood cell count > 16,000 per $mm^3$
- Blood glucose > 200 mg/dL
- Serum lactate dehydrogenase > 350 U/L
- AST > 250 U/L

During initial 48 hours:

- Hematocrit fall > 10 percent
- Blood urea nitrogen increase > 5 mg/dL
- Serum calcium < 8 mg/dL
- Base deficit > 4 mEq/L
- Fluid sequestration > 6,000 mL
- $PaO_2$ < 60 mm Hg
- Scoring: One point for each criterion met
    - o   If the score ≥ 3, severe pancreatitis likely.
    - o   If the score < 3, severe pancreatitis is unlikely

| Score | % Mortality |
|-------|-------------|
| 0 - 2 | 2 |
| 3 - 4 | 15 |
| 5 - 6 | 40 |
| 7 - 8 | 100 |

# Revised Cardiac Risk Index

Revised cardiac risk index

- High-risk type of surgery (intraperitoneal, intrathoracic, or suprainguinal vascular surgery)
- History of ischemic heart disease
- History of CHF
- History of cerebrovascular disease
- Diabetes mellitus requiring treatment with insulin
- Preoperative serum creatinine > 2.0 mg/dL

| Risk factors | Cardiac Risk (%) |
|:---:|:---:|
| 0 | 0.4 |
| 1 | 1.0 |
| 2 | 2.4 |
| 3 or more | 5.4 |

# My notes

Sunita Sharma MD, PhD

# My notes

My notes

# My notes

# My notes

# My notes

# Important Pagers

# Abbreviations

AAA Abdominal Aortic Aneurysm

ABG Arterial Blood Gas

AMA Against Medical Advice

ATN Acute Tubular Necrosis

BID Two times a day

BMI Body Mass Index

BP Blood Pressure

BUN Blood Urea Nitrogen

CAD Coronary Artery Disease

CBC Complete Blood Count

COPD Chronic Obstructive Pulmonary Disease

CT Computerized Tomography

CXR Chest X-Ray

DBP Diastolic Blood Pressure

DIC Disseminated Intravascular Coagulation

DKA Diabetic Ketoacidosis

EEG Electroencephalogram

EF Ejection Fraction

EKG Electrocardiogram

GERD Gastroesophageal Reflux Disease

IM Intramuscular

IV Intravenous

NPO Nothing orally

# Abbreviations

NSAID Non Steroidal Anti-inflammatory Drug

OT Occupational Therapy

PICC Peripherally Inserted Central Catheter

PO Per Oral

PRN As needed

PT Physical Therapy

Q4H Every four hours

Q6H Every six hours

QHS At bed time

QID Four times a day

RRT Rapid Response Team

SBP Systolic Blood Pressure

TID Three times a day

TSH Thyroid Stimulating Hormone

# Index

# Index

www.ingramcontent.com/pod-product-compliance
Lightning Source LLC
Chambersburg PA
CBHW022130170526
45157CB00004B/1827